High Performance Living

Take Charge of Your Destiny

Table of Contents

The only way to do great work is to love what you do. If you haven't found it yet, keep looking. Don't settle. As with all matters of the heart, you'll know when you find it. And, like any great relationship, it just gets better and better as the years roll on.

— Steve Jobs

Chapter 1. Introduction

Prepare to embark on a transformative journey toward peak living with our Special Report titled "High Performance Living: Take Charge of Your Destiny." This isn't just a guide, but an engaging opportunity to revitalize your life - mentally, physically, and spiritually. Its enlightening insights might be all you need to wake up every morning with renewed vigor, navigate your everyday with enviable stamina, and end your days fulfilled. Be it rebooting your: health, reviving relationships, amplifying productivity, or enhancing personal happiness—our Special Report covers all. An uncompromised life awaits, all you need is to make a choice. So, if you're ready to seize your destiny, embracing your potential to live at highest, let's dive in! After all, the most wonderful journey you can take is the one within yourself.

Chapter 2. Understanding the Foundations of High Performance Living

High performance living is not merely about being productive and efficient at what we do; rather, it encompasses a holistic approach to life that prioritizes excellence in all areas. It calls for a commitment to continuous improvement – from our professional careers to personal relationships, from our physical health to our mental well-being. The pursuit of high performance requires robust foundations that can stand the test of time, challenging circumstances, and changing environments.

2.1. Establishing the Key Pillars

High performance living is founded upon four key pillars — Health, Relationships, Productivity, and Personal Happiness. It is these pillars that offer the requisite support and strength throughout our high performance journey.

Health, the first pillar, not only refers to physical well-being but also to mental and emotional wellness. It is having the strength and stamina necessary to withstand the pressures and demands of daily life. Furthermore, good health allows us to engage fully in every facet of our lives, from work to hobbies to personal relationships.

The second pillar, relationships, reflects our connections with other people. Relationships provide a sense of belonging and purpose; they are a source of joy, comfort, support, and love. High performers value and actively cultivate positive and enriching relationships in their lives.

Productivity, our third pillar, transcends mere task completion. It encompasses the effective use of our time, energy, talents, and resources to create maximum impact. High performers aren't just busy; they strategically work towards their goals, prioritizing activities that move them closer to their desired outcomes.

Lastly, Personal Happiness, the fourth pillar, plays a vital role. High performers consider enjoyment and fulfillment as an integral part of their journey, not just the destination. They comprehend that true success transcends material achievement and includes emotional well-being and inner peace.

2.2. The Crucial Role of Self-Belief

Self-belief is a crucial element in high performance living. It is the firm conviction in one's abilities, the deep-rooted confidence that whatever comes, one has the skills and mindset to emerge victorious. High performers have absolute trust in their abilities, and they use this belief as a fuel to motivate, inspire and guide them on their journey toward peak performance.

Building self-belief is a continuous and dynamic process. It involves rebuilding and fortifying yourself after setbacks, learning from failures, and celebrating victories – no matter how small.

2.3. Cultivation of Resilience

Succeeding in the realm of high performance living necessitates the cultivation of resilience. Resilience is the ability to persevere and remain steadfast in the face of adversity, to bend but not break under pressure, and to rebound with renewed determination after a setback. It equips high performers with the tenacity to stay on course, surmount challenges, and continue their journey towards peak performance.

Resilience is closely interwoven with emotional intelligence, which is the capacity to understand, process, and manage own as well as others' emotions. It equips high performers with the ability to maintain a balanced and optimistic outlook, even in the face of rigorous demands and challenging situations.

2.4. The Power of Mindset

Having the right mindset is another significant facet of high performance living. A positive, growth-oriented mindset propels high performers towards their goals, instigating them to learn, grow, and strive for excellence. They understand that success is not a destination, but a journey defined by constant learning and improvement.

High performers also acknowledge the importance of a 'success mindset' – a belief system that supports their aspirations and objectives. This includes elements like ambition, optimism, persistence, resilience, adaptability, and an insatiable desire to better oneself.

2.5. Developing Consistent and Effective Habits

High performers recognize that their habits constitute an integral part of their journey. The consistent, daily actions performed intentionally and deliberately contribute significantly to their success. Seemingly small habits culminate to create big results over time.

Understanding and implementing the principles of habit formation and habit change are vital. High performers perceive habits as a path to mastery and are mindful in their choice of habits, ensuring they align with their higher purposes and closer towards achieving their goals.

2.6. Spirituality and High Performance Living

No discussion of high performance living can be complete without incorporating spirituality. High performers perceive spirituality as the inner compass guiding them towards their highest potential. It imbues their journey with purpose and direction, fostering a sense of connection with the universe and their unique role within it.

In summary, high performance living thrives on a sturdy foundation that incorporates health, relationships, productivity and personal happiness as its pillars. It demands self-belief, resilience, a growth-oriented mindset, effective habits, and spiritual anchoring. As you journey towards achieving high performance in all facets of your life, understanding these foundations will equip you to create a life of fulfilling achievement and deep inner satisfaction. Remember the journey is as important, if not more, than the destination. May the path towards high performance living pave your way to a life of joyous fulfillment, unwavering success, and deep-rooted happiness.

Chapter 3. Revitalizing Health: Fitness, Nutrition, and Mental Tenacity

The pursuit of health is a central tenet in high-performance living; it is the platform from which we launch all our other endeavors. A healthy existence is not limited to just our physical being, but includes a robust mental state as well. This chapter will unmask the ultimate trifecta of a high-performance life: fitness, nutrition, and mental tenacity, culminating in a comprehensive, multidimensional approach to health.

3.1. Fitness: The Physical Foundation of High-performance

Fitness is a key enabler of an achieving lifestyle with numerous benefits such as optimizing cardiovascular health, maintaining healthy weight, enhancing mood, and boosting energy levels. It's crucial to partake in regular, structured movement, choosing activities that are both enjoyable and challenging.

Regardless of one's starting point, embarking on a fitness journey involves mapping an individualized route towards the desired endpoint. Small, consistent steps bring us closer to reaching this goal, ensuring that our fitness regimen becomes a sustainable part of our lifestyle.

1. aerobic exercises (such as running, biking, and swimming) to strengthen the cardiovascular system

2. resistance training to build and maintain muscle mass

3. flexibility and balance exercises to enhance mobility and

decrease the risk of injury

It's essential to remember the principle of progressive overload, stating that in order to grow stronger and more resilient, our bodies need to be habitually exposed to training demands above the existing capacity. This way, our bodies are compelled to adapt to the increased load, resulting in improved strength and endurance.

3.2. Nutrition: Fuel for a High-performance Life

The quality of the fuel we give our bodies profoundly influences performance. To function at peak capacity, we require quality sources of macronutrients (proteins, carbohydrates, and fats), as well as a wide scope of micronutrients (vitamins and minerals).

A clean, nutrient-dense diet can launch our bodies towards optimum performance. It's crucial to consume:

1. proteins to build and repair muscles

2. complex carbohydrates to provide a sustained energy source

3. healthy fats to support satiety, brain function, and absorption of fat-soluble vitamins

4. an ample array of fruits and vegetables to ensure a plentiful supply of fiber, vitamins, and antioxidants

Refined and processed foods, along with excessive sugar intake, should be kept to a bare minimum, due to their potential negative impact on both physical health and cognitive prowess. Hydration is also key - not only for maintaining bodily functions, but also for optimizing cognitive abilities.

3.3. Mental Tenacity: The Bedrock of High-performance

The mind is an influential player in the high-performance game. Just as the body needs regular training to stay fit, the mind demands continual nurturing to sustain a high level of function. It's essentially about developing and strengthening cognitive resilience, creating enhanced endurance against the various challenges life throws at us.

Mindfulness practice such as meditation is shown to improve cognitive function and stress management. Regularly detaching from our incessant work or task-oriented thoughts promotes mental recovery, making space for increased productivity and creativity. The coupling of mindfulness with positive psychology practices like gratitude journaling, can significantly contribute to boosting our mental tenacity.

Physical exercise also substantially contributes to our mental fortitude. The release of 'feel-good hormones' during and after exercise can lift mood and act as a natural antidote to stress, anxiety, and depression.

Essentially, optimum health is achievable as long as we place equal importance on physical fitness, nutritional sustenance, and mental resilience. When all these realms are given the attention they deserve, we position ourselves on the launching pad: ready to propel towards the highest zones of performance and success. The journey of revitalizing health is a transformative one and requires total commitment and patience. However, the rewards are profound, granting us not only a healthier existence but a fortified platform from which we can leap towards our highest achievable destiny.

Remember, every step towards a healthier life is a step towards a higher-performance life. It's time to seize the resources offered in this chapter and take the reins of your health, steering your life towards unimagined summits of performance and satisfaction. The journey towards high performance is an active pursuit – a quest of continuous growth, resilience, and exhilaration. Let this chapter be your guideline, your light in the pathway to self-discovery and attaining peak performance.

Chapter 4. Enhancing Personal Relationships: A Key Pillar of a High-performance Life

Humans are inherently social animals, hardwired for interactions. Subsequently, the quality of our relationships tends to have a deep-seated impact on our wellbeing, success, and overall life-performance. In building a life of high performance, taking the effort to solidify and enhance personal relationships therefore becomes not only beneficial, but integral.

4.1. The Role of Relationships in High Performance

Our first point of exploration dives into the depths of the profound correlation between relationships and human performance. Henry Ford once said, "Coming together is a beginning; keeping together is progress; working together is success." Indeed, excellent relationships provide a solid foundation, fostering personal growth and reinforcing resilience.

The echo of supporting research from the realm of social neuroscience resonates this notion, illustrating the significant role relationships play in our cognitive function, motivation, and emotional health. Furthermore, Harvard's 75-year-long Grant study determined that good relationships were the most thing people needed to be happy.

When we surround ourselves with supportive and nurturing relationships, we end up creating an environment that is conducive to our wellbeing, productivity, and growth. Quality relationships, therefore, prove to be a critical underpinning of a high-performance life, serving as a spectacular source for motivation, comfort, and inspiration.

4.2. The Art of Building and Nurturing Relationships

At its core, the art of building and nurturing relationships is about empathy, communication, and commitment. Great relationships are not necessarily devoid of conflict, but they involve effective conflict resolution built on trust and understanding.

Empathy involves understanding and sharing an individual's feelings, fostering a sense of mutual respect and understanding. Effective communication, of course, is key for expressing thoughts, feelings and concerns constructively and diplomatically. Lastly commitment emphasizes dedication to maintaining and developing the relationship, even when things get tough.

4.3. Fostering Healthy Family Relations

Family, as the basic social unit, plays a significant role in shaping individuals. Consequently, maintaining healthy family relations is critical to harness positivity and provide a platform for emotional growth. Healthy family relationships serve as safe havens, providing support, comfort and unconditional love.

Communication is The epicenter of all healthy relationships. Encouraging open dialogues, active listening, expressing feelings with respect and consideration, can all help to foster connecting bridges, mending any cracks that might exist.

4.4. Thriving in Romantic Relationships

As with family, romantic relationships can also significantly impact wellbeing and performance. Harmony in such relationships can enhance mental health, foster better stress management, and even boost immune function.

To nurture a flourishing romantic relationship, practice appreciation and respect. Frequent expressions of love, gratitude, and admiration contribute in creating positive bonding experiences. Moreover, ensuring equality in decisions and sharing responsibilities builds respect and a sense of partnership.

4.5. Creating Strong Social Connections

Beyond the immediate bonds of family and romance, we must not overlook the importance of social connections. Friends, colleagues, and even casual acquaintances can enrich our lives immensely, providing avenues for relaxation, shared interests, and mutual support.

Fostering and maintaining these connections often require intentional efforts and time commitment. Regular communication, sharing experiences, and showing support during tough times can help in creating bonds that last.

4.6. Dealing with Relationship Challenges

Life is an unpredictable series of ebbs and flows, and relationships have their fair share. Addressing relationship challenges head-on, with patience and understanding, can be the key to turning these difficulties into opportunities for growth. This involves practicing empathy, understanding, patience, and consistently striving for open and honest communication. Remember: every relationship has its difficulties but overcoming them in a constructive manner is what sets high-performing relationships apart.

4.7. The Road Ahead: Continual Relationship Enhancement

The journey of high performance is a never-ending path of growth. Similarly, the pursuit of stronger and better relationships is a continuous process that requires lifelong commitment. Whether it's becoming more empathetic, improving your communication skills or finding ways to show your appreciation, there's always room for improvement. Remember, growth in relationships reflects growth in life, hence continuous enhancement is a key pillar of a high-performance life.

This chapter has offered the start of the roadmap to enhancing personal relationships, a cornerstone in the journey towards high performance living. Starting from understanding the prime role that effective relationships play, we dove into the skills and attitudes required to form and nourish them, along with ways to handle challenges that could arise. As we hold these insights, we continue our odyssey, understanding that enhancing our relationships is a revolving process of learning, adjusting, and growing. Looking at the grand panorama of life, at the end of the day, all we are left with are the relationships we cherished and nurtured. They are the true epitome of a high-performance life. With this consciousness, let us perpetually strive to make our personal relationships better, enriching every single day, and indeed, enhancing our lives.

Chapter 5. Productivity Amplifiers: Tools and Techniques for Peak Performance

As we delve into the realm of high performance living, it's essential to focus on productivity amplifiers, namely the tools and techniques that fuel peak performance.

5.1. Unleashing Potential with Right Tools

Imagine you are an artisan in a complex age of productivity. Your craft is your life's work and to perfect it, you require the right tools instrumental in drawing out your true potential. In our context, these tools are digital and analog implements that help you manage your tasks more effectively, thereby freeing up more time and mental energy for creative and strategic thinking.

Digital tools can range from simple apps for organizing to-do lists to comprehensive software for project management. From popular picks such as Evernote for note-taking, Trello for task-tracking, Google Drive for document collaboration and storage, to more in-depth tools like Asana for project management, the right digital shortcut can convert chaotic workstreams into an organized symphony of productivity.

By contrast, the realm of analog tools revels in the tactile experience it provides. These include traditional note-taking method, bullet journals that divide your goals into digestible tasks, a simple physical calendar to block time for projects or even a whiteboard wall for brainstorming. These tools stand their ground in today's technology-driven world because they cater to those who relish the physical act of writing and conceptualizing ideas in a spatial format.

5.2. Techniques to Streamline Productivity

The tools you decide to wield are one side of the coin. The other half is the assembly of techniques, routines and practices that streamline your productivity. Please note that no technique should be considered universally applicable - what may work wonders for one individual might not be optimal for another.

One such technique is the 'Pomodoro Technique', which advocates for 25-minute bursts of focused work, followed by short breaks. Over time, this trains your mind to focus more intensely, and the breaks refresh the brain, leading to sustained productivity.

Another tactic revolves around time blocking, which is as simple as it sounds: assigning blocks of time to specific tasks or themes. This strategy can help guard against context-switching, which can be draining and disrupts momentum.

The 'Eisenhower Matrix' is a popular productivity strategy that sorts tasks into four quadrants based on their urgency and importance. This methodology helps prioritize time and energy on tasks that matter most.

The '2-Minute Rule' is another gem. If a task will take two minutes or less to complete, then do it right away instead of pushing it to your to-do list. This technique works well in tandem with time-blocking, facilitating tidying up miscellaneous tasks quickly and efficiently.

The '80/20 Rule' or 'Pareto Principle' states that 80 percent of outcomes come from 20 percent of causes. When applied to productivity, it can be interpreted as focusing on the 20 percent of your activities that produce 80 percent of your results. This approach is vital in directing your efforts where they'll be most impactful.

Remember, maintaining a high-productivity routine isn't about packing as many tasks as possible into your day. It's about selecting strategies that allow you to accomplish your key tasks in the most efficient way, to free up time, and mental energy for the activities that truly enrich your life.

5.3. Balancing Productivity and Performance

Achieving peak performance requires optimizing productivity, but it doesn't imply constant busyness. True productivity is about doing more of what matters and less of what doesn't. It means being focused on what you want to achieve, which direction you want to move in, and deciding what trade-offs make sense for you.

Keeping an eye on balance is crucial as without a work-life boundary, the chase for productivity can lead to burnout. Hence, it's essential to inject downtime into your schedule for activities that rejuvenate and support your overall well-being.

The art and science of productivity are complex and continually evolving. But taking the time to explore, experiment, and find what works best for you can empower your journey towards high performance living. By selecting the right tools and techniques to manage your time, energy, and focus, you're setting the stage for your best work - and life - yet.

Remember, the frontiers of productivity continue to expand, and evolve with each individual. So, start your journey, experiment with tools and techniques, learn from your experience, and create the customized toolbox which catapults you towards your high-performance life.

Chapter 6. Emotional Intelligence: The Unseen Facet of High Performance

Emotional intelligence, often overshadowed by its cognitive counterpart, plays an indispensable role in the construct of high performance living. Reflected in an individual's abilities to perceive, express, understand, and manage emotions, it serves as the unseen engine driving enhanced interpersonal relationships, improved decision-making, and amplified motivation, key components that define an individual's capacity to perform at their highest.

6.1. Decoding Emotional Intelligence

Emotional intelligence, a term popularised by psychologist Daniel Goleman, can be dissected into five fundamental components:

1. Self-awareness: This refers to an individual's capacity to recognize one's own emotions and how they impact thoughts and behaviors. Awareness of one's strengths and weaknesses aids in building the self-confidence required for high performance.

2. Self-regulation: Self-regulation is the ability to control intrusive or impulsive responses to emotional stimuli. It allows an individual to pivot with adaptability and flexibility, seamlessly navigating through change — a trait indispensable in enhancing life quality and productivity.

3. Motivation: This represents an inner drive and passion that transcends superficial rewards such as fame and recognition. It propels individuals toward goals and catalyzes personal satisfaction and fulfillment.

4. Empathy: Empathy is the sensitivity to interpret other people's emotions and reciprocate appropriate responses. It strengthens the bonds of interpersonal relationships, indispensable in the realm of high-performance living.

5. Social Skills: Effective communication, conflict management, and the direction of positive influences are a part of this integral component. Mastering social skills enables harmonious interactions, fostering a fertile social environment for growth and success.

Understanding these elements is the first step towards comprehending the vast landscape of emotional intelligence and its critical role in a high-performance life.

6.2. The Power of Emotional Intelligence

Emotional intelligence plays an enormous role in exploiting our full potential and, in turn, maximizing our performance. It bridges the gap between knowing and doing, translating knowledge into actionable steps leading to success.

1. Decision-Making: Emotionally intelligent individuals comprehend the emotional drivers of their actions. This understanding leads to effective decision-making, propelled by rational thought, not whims of transitory emotion.

2. Relationships: Emotional intelligence equips individuals with the tools to understand, communicate, and resolve. This fosters bonds, highlighting its role in successful personal and professional relationships.

3. Health: Emotional intelligence can impact physical and mental health. It equips you to manage stress effectively, staving off potential health complications like hypertension, heart disease, and anxiety disorders.

4. Performance: Studies correlate high emotional intelligence with optimal performance, especially in leadership roles. It helps in tackling stressful situations, conflict resolution, and team dynamics, all leading to improved productivity.

Tapping into the power of emotional intelligence can dramatically elevate an individual's performance, thus enriching different life aspects.

6.3. Enhancing Emotional Intelligence: Techniques and Practices

Cultivating emotional intelligence is a continuous task, requiring constant self-reflection, patience, and practice. A few techniques and practices include:

1. Mindfulness Meditation: Regular practice of mindfulness meditation can enhance self-awareness and self-regulation. It facilitates emotional balance and fosters mental clarity, integral aspects of emotional intelligence.

2. Journaling: Penning down thoughts can help in understanding emotions better, leading to improved self-awareness and regulation. It serves as a tool of introspection and aids in emotional growth.

3. Empathic Listening: Cultivating the habit of empathic listening can improve empathy and social skills. It involves understanding the emotions and perspectives of others without any judgment or interruption, enhancing the quality of interpersonal relationships.

4. Emotional Literacy: Identifying and labeling emotions correctly is an essential step in developing emotional intelligence.

5. Seek Feedback: To apprehend the areas of improvement, one

should seek feedback from peers, mentors, or family members who can provide unbiased insights about our behaviors and emotional responses.

Emotional intelligence, the unseen facet of high performance, can be fortified using these practical methods, ultimately emboldening individuals to live a high-performance life.

6.4. Emotional Intelligence and Resilience: Bonds of Steel

Resilience, the ability to bounce back from adversities, is fundamentally linked to emotional intelligence—both are reliant on self-awareness, regulation, and the ability to maintain emotional equilibrium.

Emotionally intelligent people synchronize their emotions and thoughts brilliantly, letting them navigate through adversities without being overwhelmed. Superior resilience allows such individuals to view failures as stepping stones, not setbacks, further bolstering their capacity to perform at peak.

At the core, the role of emotional intelligence in nurturing resilience provides the sustainability factor in high performance living, enabling one to constantly perform, evolve, and triumph over obstacles without fizzling out in the long term.

Understanding emotional intelligence, its components, its power, the techniques to enhance it, and its relation with resilience provides a comprehensive view of this unseen facet integral for a high-performance life. Harnessing its potential can unlock an unimagined version of yourself, optimized for success, happiness, and fulfillment. Finally, remember that emotional intelligence, as with any other skill, improves with practice-myriad opportunities await you each day to learn, adapt, and improve.

Chapter 7. Creating a High-performance Mindset: Strategies and Frameworks

Creating a high-performance mindset is essential to reaching the peak of your potentials and truly taking charge of your destiny. This chapter dives into the strategies and frameworks necessary to cultivate this mindset, equipping you with insights on mental fortitude, embracing challenges, and harnessing your cognitive and emotional intelligence.

7.1. Embracing Challenges and Developing Mental Fortitude

To trace the path towards a high-performance mindset, we first need to understand the importance of embracing challenges. Challenges are like crucibles that temper the mind, making it stronger, flexible, and more resilient. They compel us to venture into the unknown, pushing our comfort zones, and teaching us invaluable lessons along the way. The first strategy to cultivate a high-performance mindset is, therefore, to willingly accept and face challenges, rather than avoiding them.

Boosting mental fortitude is a demonstrable trait of high-performers. It is the persistent and consistent determination to carry on despite setbacks and failures. Mental fortitude isn't about never falling; it's about getting back up every time you fall. Embracing failure as an opportunity for growth and learning is, thus, a stepping stone on your path to a high-performance mindset.

7.2. Harnessing Cognitive and Emotional Intelligence

The second key strategy focuses on developing cognitive and emotional intelligence. Cognitive intelligence includes the skills we use to learn, analyze, understand, reason, and draw conclusions based on our experiences. High cognitive intelligence correlates with improved decision-making abilities, problem-solving skills, and learning capacity, all crucial to high performance.

Emotional intelligence, on the other hand, relates to our ability to understand, interpret, and respond to our own and others' emotions. More than just empathy, it includes aspects of self-awareness, emotional regulation, motivation, and social skills. When harnessed appropriately, emotional intelligence can fuel resilience, effective leadership, and positive relationships, all crucial building blocks of a high-performance mindset.

7.3. Building a Growth Mindset

One of the most effective ways to navigate towards a high-performance mindset is by cultivating a growth mindset—a belief that abilities can be nurtured and intelligence honed with focused effort. Unlike a fixed mindset, which perceives intelligence and abilities as inherent and unchangeable, a growth mindset relishes challenges, embraces failures as learning opportunities, and manifests more resilience, thereby paving the way to high performance.

7.4. The Role of Visualization and Affirmations

Visualizing your success involves imagining yourself achieving your goals. This mental rehearsal primes your mind to act according to your visions, influencing both conscious and subconscious actions. Coupled with positive affirmations—proactively stating and affirming your abilities—it creates a rewarding feedback loop that boosts self-confidence and helps to form a high-performance mindset.

7.5. Implementing the Four C's Framework

An effective structure to underpin these strategies is the Four C's Framework—Consistency, Challenge, Confidence, Control. Consistency underlines the importance of regular practice, creating strong neural pathways and habits along the path to a high-performance lifestyle. Challenge emphasizes the need to stretch one's abilities, thereby fostering growth. Confidence relates to fostering self-belief, boosted by successfully navigating through challenges. Lastly, Control underscores the capacity to influence one's life direction, reinforcing autonomy and influencing outcomes—a quintessential trait of a high-performance mindset.

In the grand scheme of things, a high-performance mindset is not a single point of achievement but a continual process of learning, growing, and adapting. It's about grit, mental fortitude, resilience, and the ability to rise in face of adversity. It involves a harmonious blend of cognitive and emotional intelligence, nurtured by a growth mindset, and underpinned by strategies such as visualization, affirmations, and the Four C's Framework. By employing these strategies, you prime yourself to reach your finest potential, empowering you to live a high-performance life and truly take charge of your destiny.

Chapter 8. Embracing Spirituality in High Performance Living

The concept of spirituality is often regarded as nebulous and abstract, yet it holds profound concrete implications for high-performance living. It becomes the grounding force that boosts mental tranquility, fosters holistic well-being, and enhances productivity. It is about recognizing our intrinsic connection to a greater universe and harnessing that understanding to achieve impressive levels of efficiency and balance in our life.

8.1. The Intricate Bond Between Spirituality and High Performance

Spirituality in high-performance living is not about religious beliefs or specific rituals. Rather, it's about cultivating a deeper sense of one's self, discovering purpose, fostering universal connectedness, and harnessing this enriched perspective for superior standards of working and living.

This sense of spirituality instills a sense of coherence and meaning to our existence. It can guide our actions, influence our decisions, and light the path towards the peak levels of performance. Strong spiritual well-being typically correlates with healthy coping mechanisms, resilience, lower levels of stress and anxiety, and improved mental health. All these contribute significantly towards a high-performance lifestyle.

Moreover, the tranquility gained through spiritual practices can help us become more focused, creative, and innovative—traits essential to high performing individuals. The positive outlook, emotional stability, and the serene mental state fostered via spiritual practices often translate into improved productivity and performance.

8.2. Incorporating Spirituality into Everyday Life

Understanding the implications of spirituality for high-performance living is just the initial step. The next crucial step is to consciously incorporate it into our daily life. Each one of us has a unique spiritual journey; there's no one-size-fits-all approach. However, certain universal strategies can help guide this journey.

1. **Mindfulness and Meditation:** These practices offer an accessible entry point to spirituality. Regular mindfulness exercises and meditation can enhance our awareness, focus, emotional balance, and well-being—key aspects critical to high performance.

2. **Nature Connection:** Regularly spending time in nature can nurture a sense of belonging to the world, fostering spiritual growth. Nature can act as a medium to free us from the constraints of our ego, helping us gain a broader perspective on life which is crucial for a high-performance lifestyle.

3. **Personal Reflection and Introspection:** Regular periods of silence, self-reflection and introspection enable us to contemplate our deeper purpose, align our actions with our values, and foster empathy—essentials for high-performance living.

4. **Being Present:** Practicing presence—immersion in the here and now—helps minimize distractions, reduces stress, and increases productivity, ensuring a high-performance lifestyle.

5. **Cultivating Positive Relationships:** Kindness, compassion, and understanding—core spiritual values—when invested in our relationships, can create supportive environments that are essential for high performance.

8.3. An Ongoing Journey - Continuous Spiritual Growth

Embracing spirituality in the quest for high-performance living is not a finite endeavor but an ongoing journey. It's an evolving process continually adapting to our changing circumstances, offering different insights at various life stages, and molding our perspective towards our pursuit of high performance.

Maintaining a spiritual diary can be an effective way to track your experiential insights and spiritual evolution. This diary can serve as your personal guide, reminding you of the broader perspective when the journey gets tough, bringing you back to your core spiritual principles, and enabling you to maintain a high-performance lifestyle.

Stand alert against turning this spiritual exploration into yet another item on your performance checklist. Rather, allow it to naturally infuse into your life, subtly influencing your thoughts, decisions, and actions. Consider this spiritual journey as a gentle but potent guidance system that progressively leads you towards the zenith of high performance.

In conclusion, spirituality forms a key component in the tapestry of high-performance living, often ignored in the hustle-bustle of our fast-paced lives. Yet, it is in quiet contemplation, in the tranquility of nature, in the deepest relationships, and in the solitude of introspection, where we can truly find ourselves, and in turn, our highest performance. Embrace the spirituality journey, and get one step closer to living your best life.

Chapter 9. Transformative Habits of High Performers

In the objective pursuit of high performance, understanding the transformative habits of highly successful and productive individuals provides an essential cornerstone upon which we can build our personal and professional growth. From time management to resilience, regular exercise to meditation, these habits form the pillars of high-performance living.

9.1. The Power of Routine

High performers thrive on routine. They understand the significance of consistency in weaving the fabric of success. They do not relegate their tasks to chance but plan them strategically, ensuring they commit to what really matters. Having a routine frees their mind from the counterproductive distractions of having to make minor decisions throughout the day. They also understand the value of flexibility within routines, allowing for unexpected situations.

9.2. Resilience and the Art of Bouncing Back

Stoicism, persistence, and resilience are primary ingredients in the secret sauce of high performers. Life will inevitably throw curveballs, but they stand firm, recover swiftly, and adapt effectively. They understand that failures are not dead ends but mere detours on the course to success and growth. This perspective allows them to see every challenge as a learning opportunity and not as an impasse.

9.3. Physical Health, Mental Wealth

For high performers, physical fitness is not an afterthought but a focal point. Regular exercise is a transformative habit that not only boosts physical health but also invigorates the mind, enhancing cognitive function and promoting emotional well-being. Healthy eating habits, regular sleep, and hydration round off their physical care regimen, enabling them to acquire and maintain the vitality required for high-performance living.

9.4. Continuous Learning: Staying Relevant

High performers have an insatiable appetite for learning. They engage in continuous growth and education, both formally and informally, understanding that knowledge is a powerful tool to navigate life's landscapes. Through reading, courses, workshops, and mentorship, they absorb varied perspectives and learn new skills, thus keeping their mental faculties sharp and adaptable.

9.5. The Art of Mindfulness

High performers understand the power of being in the 'now.' They practice mindfulness, which imbues them with a deeper sense of connection to their actions, thoughts, and feelings. By staying present, they reduce anxiety, enhance focus, and maximize their potential at any given moment. This could involve meditative practices, yoga, or simply, conscious immersion in their daily tasks.

9.6. The Time Management Matrix

High performers master the science and art of managing their most precious commodity—time. They understand where to invest and when to withhold their time and effort. From Eisenhower's Time Management Matrix to the Pareto Principle, they employ strategic frameworks to categorize tasks based on their urgency and importance. This results in their remarkable productivity and effectiveness.

9.7. Building Strong Relationships

High-performance living requires human connection and strong networks. High performers recognize this and invest time and effort to cultivate impactful relationships. They appreciate the might of emotional intelligence in dealing with people, navigating conflicts, and building trust. Importantly, they understand that relationships are not just for the good times; they are the support systems aiding them during challenging periods.

9.8. Setting and Pursuing Achievable Goals

High performers are practical dreamers. They envision grand goals but break them down into achievable milestones. This process allows them to avoid overwhelm while keeping their eyes on the ultimate prize. They blend ambition with realism, creating a blend that propels them forward without inducing burnout.

By embracing the transformative habits of high performers, we can empower ourselves to lead a high-performance life. Remember, these habits are not ingrained overnight. It involves consistent effort, unyielding determination, and the courage to challenge one's limitations. Start by incorporating one habit at a time, see the life-altering transformations unfold, and ultimately, take charge of your destiny with full command.

Chapter 10. Overcoming Life Challenges: Resilience and Perseverance

Life invariably presents us with trials and tribulations that have the potential to knock us off our stride and hinder our quest for high performance living. Whether it's a sudden shift in our personal circumstances, job loss, health issues, or the loss of a loved one, life's chaos can test our strength and resilience. At these moments, it's paramount to understand and foster the innate powers of resilience and perseverance that can help us overcome these challenges and propel us forward toward our destiny.

10.1. Defining Resilience

Resilience can be conceptualized as our inner capacity to adapt effectively in the face of adversity, bounce back from difficulties, and even grow during and following substantial stress. It includes our potential to process challenging experiences and remain committed to our goals without losing our sense of self or inner stability. Resilience does not mean the absence of difficulties, but rather, it indicates our ability to tackle them head-on and come out stronger than before.

10.2. Harnessing the Power of Resilience

To harness the power of resilience, it's crucial to maintain a balanced and realistic outlook on life. Adversity will come, but effectively managing our thoughts and emotions can equip us with the fortitude to navigate such testing times. Scientific research suggests the importance of maintaining positive emotions, even during stress. These positive emotions can broaden our perspective and enable more flexible thinking, ultimately enhancing our problem-solving abilities and allowing for more effective coping strategies.

Also key to resilience is cultivating an unshakeable belief in your abilities. Such self-confidence can serve as a protective shield, safeguarding your wellbeing and propelling you through life's obstacles. Furthermore, always remember that it's alright to seek help when you need it. Strong support networks, which can include family, friends, or professionals, can provide us with needed perspective and guidance, contributing to our reservoir of resilience.

10.3. Understanding the Nature of Perseverance

Perseverance, the steadfast persistence in pursuing a course of action despite challenges, difficulties, or discouragement, is another vital companion in your journey toward high performance living. Perseverance is not about never failing or falling, but rather about continually rising each time we fall. It couples with resilience, empowering us to withstand and move forward through life's adversities.

10.4. The Art of Perseverance

The art of fostering perseverance revolves around steadfast commitment to one's goals, regardless of the hurdles that may crop up along the path. Such commitment necessitates an understanding of why your goals matter, and tying these reasons to your personal identity can keep that motivational flame burning even when times get tough.

Further, it's crucial to break our larger goals into smaller, manageable tasks. Accomplishing each of these small tasks infuses us with a sense of achievement and satisfaction that fuels our motivation for future tasks. This process of progressive mastery not only pushes us along our chosen path but also strengthens our resilience by cementing our confidence in our abilities to overcome adversity.

Additionally, being adaptable is essential. While single-minded focus on our objectives is important, adaptability permits us to readjust our sails when circumstances shift. This adaptability can help diminish potential disillusionment, frustration, or burnout, ensuring the longevity of our perseverance.

10.5. Resilience and Perseverance in the Context of High Performance Living

When resilience and perseverance are incorporated into our lives, they act as a driving force that empowers us to effectively manage and overcome life's challenges. Embracing these abilities encourages emotional balance, enhances well-being, and ultimately, facilitates a life of high performance.

Optimizing these virtues requires persistent practice, as well as the cultivation of self-awareness, emotional intelligence, and healthy coping mechanisms. Pushing through adversity rather than avoiding it hardens our resilience, fosters our perseverance, and carves the path for us to lead a life of superior productivity, enhanced personal relationships, and steadfast progress toward our loftiest aspirations.

By engraving resilience and perseverance into our lifestyles, we more readily navigate the unexpected gusts of life's storms and persist on our journey of high performance living. So, as we confront the tumultuous seas of life's challenges, we remain unflinching, weaving our resilience and perseverance into the fabric of our being, embodying the principles of high performance living, and surging forward on our path toward our ultimate destiny.

Chapter 11. Blueprint to Lifelong Success: Measurement, Maintenance, and Growth

Standing at the dawn of lifelong success, you are better equipped now with a handful of strategies and techniques that can help you traverse the less traveled path of high performance living. However, this is not where the road ends. Creating a blueprint for lifelong success entails a measured and continuous cycle of measurement, maintenance, and growth.

11.1. How to Measure Success

The journey begins with an assessment of where you stand today. It's important to develop metrics to evaluate your success. Your metrics could be tangible such as the number of books read per month, or intangible like the level of satisfaction in personal relationships.

The first step is to list down the areas that are important to you. Examples could be career success, mental health, physical fitness, relationships, and personal development. Once you have a list, devise a detailed and practical plan, with the help of a mentor, counselor, or life coach if needed. Your plan should include actionable steps you can take to achieve success in each of these domains.

The **SMART** (Specific, Measurable, Achievable, Relevant, and Time-bound) goal strategy can greatly assist in this process. Targets should be:

- *Specific*: Avoid vague goals and instead aim for specific targets like losing 10 pounds in three months.

- *Measurable*: Make sure you have ways to measure your progress.

- *Achievable*: Your goals should be attainable; too lofty aspirations can lead to discouragement.

- *Relevant*: Goals should be relevant to your overall life objectives and values.

- *Time-bound*: Assign a timeline to ensure that the goal has a beginning and end date.

11.2. Maintaining Success

While measuring success is essential, equally important is maintaining it. Many people witness steady progress, only to find it dwindling after a while. Consistently repeating the actions that led to initial success is necessary for maintaining it. This requires discipline, perseverance, motivation, and adaptability.

One effective method to establish discipline and consistency is through the use of habit trackers. They not only provide a visual representation of your progress but also instill a sense of satisfaction as you cross off each successful day.

Another essential aspect of maintenance is the regular review and adjustment of your goals. Life circumstances and personal changes often mandate modifications in previously set targets. Adaptability in adjusting these goals as per your current situation and aspirations is a mark of a high performer.

11.3. Embracing Growth

High performance living is a lifelong journey and not a destination. Therefore, it's vital to keep aiming for growth, even when you achieve desired success in certain areas. Building on your learning, challenging yourself, and venturing out of your comfort zone are crucial for continuous personal development.

Embracing a growth mindset—a belief that abilities and intelligence can be developed—is fundamental. People with a growth mindset are more likely to persevere in the face of adversity, see failures as opportunities for learning, and are continuously looking for ways to improve.

Reaping the benefits of lifelong learning is another path toward growth. This involves committing to continuous education and self-improvement. This could mean learning a new skill, enhancing existing ones, or expanding your knowledge base.

11.4. Conclusion

High performance living is a choice each one of us can make. It's an opportunity to transcend beyond the ordinary and unleash the extraordinary within us. It's a journey of continuous growth and self-improvement with a commitment to get better each day. The blueprint to lifelong success lays before you. Measure your progress rigorously, maintain what you have achieved, and always strive for growth. As you continue this journey, remember, high performance isn't a sprint; it's a marathon. Success is not just about crossing the finish line but also about enjoying the run, cherishing the milestones, and learning from the hurdles. So take that positive stride towards a better you, because the most rewarding journey you will ever embark on is the journey within yourself.